Ginger

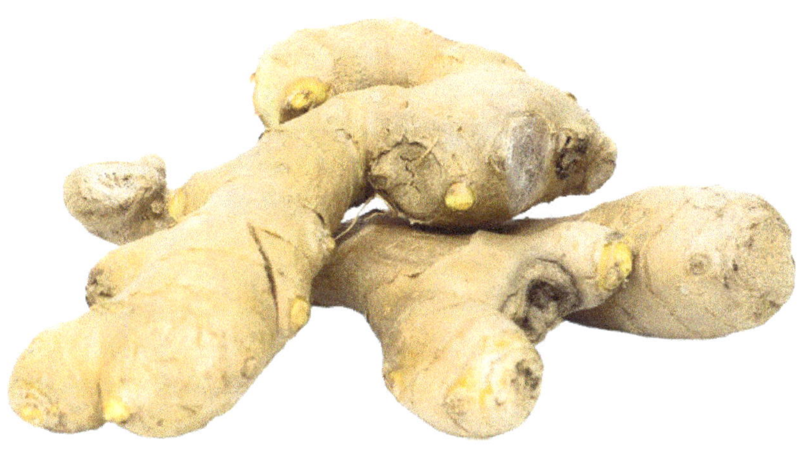

H. - G. Saenger

The Book:

The Journey into the World of Ginger

Ginger, a root with a storied history and an abundance of uses, has captivated the hearts and minds of people for centuries. As a staple in many culinary dishes and a key ingredient in traditional medicine, ginger is a beloved and versatile spice. The Book: Ginger. Unlocking the Secrets of a Powerful Root delves deep into the world of ginger, uncovering ist rich history, extensive health benefits, and various applications in our daily lives.

The Author:

H.-G. Saenger
Passionate hobby cook and
interested author, lives with his second
since 2020 with his second wife
in Thailand.

Ginger

Unlocking the Secrets of a Powerful Root

by

H. - G. Saenger

GINGER

Table of Contents:

Introduction: The Journey into the World of Ginger

Ginger, a root with a storied history and an abundance of uses, has captivated the hearts and minds of people for centuries. As a staple in many culinary dishes and a key ingredient in traditional medicine, ginger is a beloved and versatile spice. The Book: Ginger. Unlocking the Secrets of a Powerful Root delves deep into the world of ginger, uncovering is rich history, extensive health benefits, and various applications in our daily lives.

Our journey begins with the humble origins of ginger, exploring its early cultivation in ancient China and India. We trace its journey across the globe, as it made its way to the Mediterranean and then the New World. Along the way, we learn about the cultural and historical significance of ginger, from its role in traditional medicine to its inclusion in ancient rituals and ceremonies.

The exploration continues with an in-depth look at the cultivation and harvesting of ginger. Understanding the lifecycle of this powerful root will provide insight into the care and patience required to nurture it from a small seed into a mature plant. We will also delve into the world of ginger essential oil, discussing its extraction, benefits, and various uses.

As we dig deeper into the world of ginger, we uncover the many health benefits it offers. From alleviating nausea and reducing inflammation to promoting cardiovascular health and aiding digestion, ginger's multifaceted health benefits are truly astounding. We will also examine ginger's role in traditional medicine around the world, highlighting the various ways it has been used to treat ailments and promote wellness.

Ginger's versatility extends beyond its medicinal uses, as it is also a beloved ingredient in the culinary world. We will explore the unique flavor profile and spice that ginger brings to various dishes, and share innovative recipes that showcase the root's versatility. This journey will also take us through ginger-infused beverages, including teas, tonics, and cocktails, highlighting the many ways in which this powerful root can be enjoyed.

As we continue our exploration, we will uncover the ways in which ginger can be integrated into skincare and beauty treatments, providing natural remedies and enhancements for various skin concerns. The journey doesn't stop there, as we also provide guidance on how to grow ginger at home, from seed to harvest, allowing you to experience the joy of cultivating this powerful root for yourself.

Throughout our journey, we will touch on the global ginger trade, examining the economics, sustainability, and fair practices that surround this vital industry. We will also look towards the future of ginger, exploring current research, innovations, and potential applications for this powerful root in various aspects of our lives.

Our journey culminates in the „Ginger Challenge," where we encourage you to integrate ginger into your daily life, harnessing its health benefits and versatility to enhance your overall well-being.

The Ginger Chronicles: Unlocking the Secrets of a Powerful Root is your comprehensive guide to the world of ginger, offering a deep understanding of its history, uses, and potential. As you embark on this journey, we invite you to embrace the power and allure of this remarkable root, and to experience for yourself the lasting impact it can have on your health, wellness, and culture.

Chapter 1: Ginger: Origins and Historical Significance

Ginger, known scientifically as Zingiber officinale, is a flowering plant whose rhizome, or underground stem, is widely used as a spice and in traditional medicine. This chapter delves into the origins of ginger, tracing its cultivation and historical significance, and exploring its role in various ancient cultures.

1.1 Early Origins and Cultivation

The origins of ginger can be traced back to ancient China and India, where it has been cultivated for over 5,000 years. It is believed to have originated in the tropical rainforests of the Indian subcontinent and Southeast Asia. Ginger was widely used in traditional Chinese and Indian medicine and was highly valued for its medicinal and culinary properties.

In ancient China, ginger was considered a gift from the gods, and it played a central role in various religious rituals and ceremonies. It was used to warm the body, stimulate digestion, and alleviate ailments such as colds and flu. In traditional Indian Ayurvedic medicine, ginger was referred to as „Mahaaushadhi," which means „the great medicine." It was utilized to treat a wide range of conditions, including digestive disorders, inflammation, and respiratory issues.

1.2 The Spread of Ginger

Ginger's journey from the East to the West can be traced back to the ancient trade routes, specifically the Silk Road, which connected Asia to the Mediterranean region. It made its way to the Roman Empire, where it was highly valued for its medicinal properties and was used to alleviate digestive issues and treat various ailments.

After the fall of the Roman Empire, ginger's popularity persisted in Europe, where it became a highly sought-after spice during the Middle Ages. It was valued not only for its medicinal uses but also for its ability to preserve food and mask the taste of spoiled meat. Ginger was considered a luxury item, and its trade was controlled by Arab merchants, who maintained a monopoly on the spice trade.

With the discovery of the New World and the establishment of sea routes, ginger's popularity spread even further. Spanish conquistadors introduced ginger to the Caribbean, where it quickly became a staple crop. From there, it made its way to Mexico and other parts of the Americas.

1.3 Ginger in Ancient Literature and Folklore

Ginger has been mentioned in various ancient texts, including Chinese, Indian, and Arabic literature. In the Chinese book „Shennong Bencaojing," which dates back to around 2700 BCE, ginger is listed as one of the most important medicinal plants. Similarly, in the Indian epic „Mahabharata," ginger is described as a powerful healing herb.

In Arabic literature, ginger is mentioned in the „One Thousand and One Nights," where it is used as an aphrodisiac and a treatment for various ailments. The Greek physician Dioscorides also discussed ginger's medicinal properties in his work „De Materia Medica," which served as a cornerstone of pharmacology for centuries.

Ginger has been associated with various myths and folklore, often symbolizing love, passion, and prosperity. In some cultures, it was believed that planting ginger near the entrance of one's home would bring good fortune and ward off evil spirits.

1.4 The Cultural and Historical Significance of Ginger

Throughout history, ginger has held a special place in various cultures. It has been used in religious ceremonies, as a form of currency, and as a symbol of love and prosperity. Its role in traditional medicine and culinary applications has made it an indispensable part of human history.

The historical significance of ginger is evident in the way it has influenced global trade, politics, and cultural exchange. The spice trade, including ginger, played a crucial role in shaping the world as we know it today. Ginger's journey from the East to the West is a testament to the power of human curiosity and the desire to explore and connect with other cultures.

The cultural impact of ginger can also be observed in various festivals and celebrations around the world. In Japan, during the annual „Shogatsu" or New Year's celebration, ginger is used in a traditional soup called „Ozoni," believed to bring good fortune for the year ahead. In the Caribbean, ginger plays a central role in the preparation of traditional dishes and beverages during Christmas festivities.

1.5 Ginger in Art and Architecture

The influence of ginger extends beyond its culinary and medicinal uses; it has also found its way into art and architecture. In ancient China, ginger was often depicted in paintings and sculptures, symbolizing vitality and health. The beautiful, intricate patterns of ginger plants have inspired various forms of art, including textiles, ceramics, and wood carvings.

The gingerbread house, a popular holiday tradition in many Western cultures, can also be traced back to ginger's historical influence. It is believed that gingerbread houses originated in Germany during the 16th century and were inspired by the elaborate sugar sculptures that were popular during that time. The tradition of creating gingerbread houses became widespread, eventually becoming a beloved holiday activity in many parts of the world.

1.6 Conclusion

The historical significance of ginger is immense, reflecting the profound impact it has had on various aspects of human life. From its early cultivation in ancient China and India to its global spread, ginger has played a crucial role in shaping the course of history.

Throughout the centuries, ginger has been used for medicinal, culinary, and even artistic purposes, showcasing its incredible versatility and cultural importance. As we continue our journey through „The Ginger Chronicles: Unlocking the Secrets of a Powerful Root," we will delve deeper into the many facets of ginger, exploring its numerous health benefits, applications in modern medicine, and its role in our daily lives.

By understanding the rich history and cultural significance of ginger, we can appreciate the power and allure of this remarkable root, and embrace its lasting impact on our health, wellness, and culture.

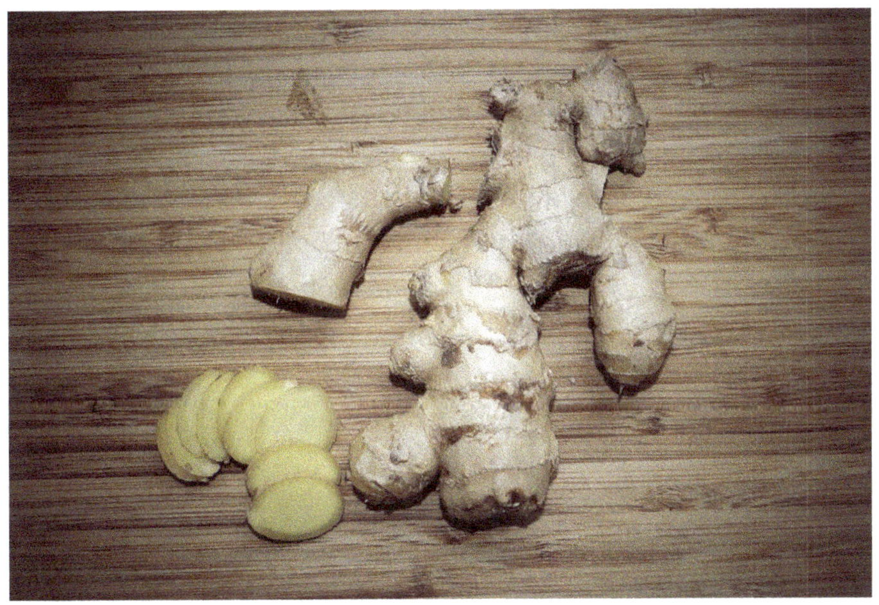

Chapter 2: Cultivation and Harvesting: The Life-cycle of Ginger

To fully appreciate the versatility and power of ginger, it is essential to understand the lifecycle of this fascinating plant. This chapter explores the cultivation and harvesting of ginger, providing insight into the care, patience, and knowledge required to nurture it from a small seed to a mature plant.

2.1 Growing Conditions and Requirements

Ginger thrives in warm, humid climates with well-draining, loamy soil. It is primarily grown in tropical and subtropical regions, with India, China, Nigeria, and Indonesia being the largest producers of ginger. The ideal temperature range for ginger cultivation is between 68°F and 86°F (20°C and 30°C), and it requires ample rainfall or irrigation to ensure steady growth.

Ginger is typically propagated using rhizome segments, known as seed pieces or „sets." These sets are cut from mature ginger rhizomes, each containing at least one viable bud or „eye." The ideal size of a seed piece is approximately 1 to 1.5 inches (2.5 to 4 cm) in length and weighing about 0.7 to 1.4 ounces (20 to 40 grams).

2.2 Planting and Cultivation

Ginger planting usually takes place during late winter or early spring when the threat of frost has passed. The seed pieces are first soaked in water for 12 to 24 hours to promote sprouting. They are then planted about 1 to 2 inches (2.5 to 5 cm) deep in well-prepared, fertile soil, with the buds facing upwards.

Ginger plants require consistent moisture, so it is important to keep the soil evenly moist throughout the growing season. Mulching can help retain moisture and regulate soil temperature. Ginger also benefits from regular applications of organic matter, such as compost or well-rotted manure, which can improve soil structure and provide essential nutrients.

The ginger plant grows upright, reaching a height of 2 to 3 feet (60 to 90 cm), with long, narrow leaves resembling those of a reed. The plant produces small, inconspicuous flowers that are usually green, yellow, or white with purple streaks.

2.3 Pest and Disease Management

Ginger plants are susceptible to various pests and diseases, which can impact their growth and yield. Common pests include aphids, spider mites, and root-knot nematodes. Diseases affecting ginger include bacterial wilt, rhizome rot, and leaf spot. To minimize the risk of pests and diseases, it is crucial to practice proper sanitation, crop rotation, and the use of disease-resistant varieties.

2.4 Harvesting Ginger

Ginger is typically harvested between 8 to 10 months after planting, depending on the intended use. Young ginger, also known as „green" or „spring" ginger, is harvested around 4 to 6 months after planting. This type of ginger has a milder flavor and tender texture, making it ideal for use in salads, stir-fries, and pickling.

Mature ginger, which is used for its robust flavor and medicinal properties, is harvested when the leaves begin to yellow and the plant starts to die back. To harvest ginger, the soil around the plant is carefully loosened, and the rhizomes are gently lifted from the ground using a garden fork or a spade. The rhizomes are then washed thoroughly to remove any remaining soil and debris.

2.5 Post-Harvest Handling and Storage

After harvesting, ginger can be used fresh or processed into various forms, such as dried, ground, or crystallized ginger. Fresh ginger can be stored in a cool, dry place for up to a month, or in the refrigerator for up to two months. To extend the shelf life of ginger, it can be stored in the freezer, either whole or grated, for up to six months.

For long-term storage, ginger can be dried or dehydrated. This process involves slicing the ginger thinly and placing the slices in a dehydrator or a low-temperature oven. Once the ginger is completely dry and brittle, it can be stored in an airtight container away from direct sunlight and moisture. Dried ginger can be ground into a powder, which is commonly used in baking, cooking, and as a dietary supplement.

Crystallized ginger, also known as candied ginger, is another popular form of preserved ginger. It is made by boiling ginger slices in a sugar syrup until they become tender and then allowing them to dry. Crystallized ginger can be enjoyed as a sweet treat or used in various recipes, such as baked goods and desserts.

2.6 Ginger Farming: Challenges and Opportunities

Ginger farming presents both challenges and opportunities for farmers around the world. The labor-intensive nature of ginger cultivation, combined with the susceptibility to pests and diseases, can make it a difficult crop to grow. However, the high demand for ginger in various industries, such as food, pharmaceuticals, and cosmetics, offers a potentially lucrative market for ginger producers.

Sustainable ginger farming practices are essential for the long-term success of the ginger industry. These practices include the use of organic fertilizers, the conservation of soil and water resources, and the adoption of integrated pest management strategies. The promotion of fair trade and ethical sourcing practices can also help ensure that ginger farmers receive fair compensation for their hard work and dedication.

2.7 Conclusion

Understanding the cultivation and harvesting process of ginger provides valuable insight into the lifecycle of this powerful root. From its early beginnings as a small seed piece to its eventual harvest, the journey of ginger is one of patience, care, and perseverance. By appreciating the effort and dedication required to cultivate and harvest ginger, we can develop a deeper respect for this remarkable plant and the many benefits it offers.

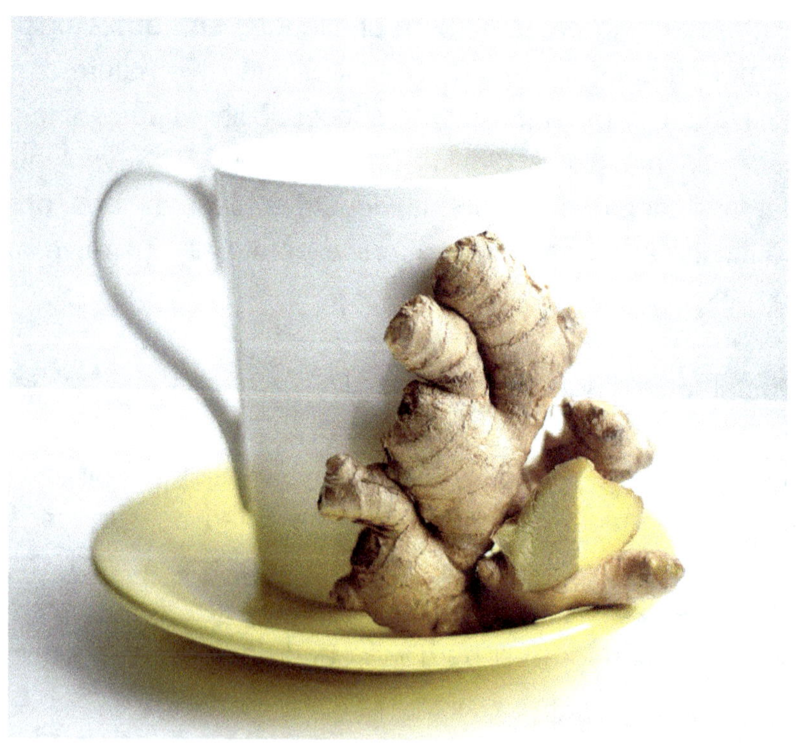

Chapter 3: Unlocking Ginger's Nutritional Profile

To truly appreciate the power and versatility of ginger, it is crucial to explore its nutritional profile. This chapter delves into the various nutrients, bioactive compounds, and antioxidants present in ginger, helping to shed light on the many health benefits and therapeutic properties associated with this potent root.

3.1 Macronutrients

Ginger is low in calories and contains a modest amount of carbohydrates, primarily in the form of dietary fiber. It contains negligible amounts of protein and fat, making it a low-energy-density food. The dietary fiber in ginger aids in digestion and contributes to feelings of satiety, which can be beneficial for those looking to maintain or lose weight.

3.2 Vitamins and Minerals

Ginger is a good source of several essential vitamins and minerals. It contains vitamin B6, which plays a crucial role in brain development and function, as well as the production of the hormones serotonin and norepinephrine, which help regulate mood. Ginger is also a source of vitamin C, an antioxidant that supports immune function and helps protect cells from damage caused by free radicals.

In terms of minerals, ginger contains small amounts of potassium, magnesium, and manganese. Potassium is vital for maintaining proper fluid balance in the body and regulating blood pressure, while magnesium is necessary for muscle function, nerve function, and energy production. Manganese is an essential trace element that plays a role in bone health, metabolism, and antioxidant activity.

3.3 Bioactive Compounds

One of the most remarkable aspects of ginger's nutritional profile is its abundance of bioactive compounds. These compounds, also known as phytochemicals, have potent antioxidant, anti-inflammatory, and therapeutic properties that contribute to the many health benefits associated with ginger.

The primary bioactive compound found in ginger is gingerol, which is responsible for ginger's characteristic pungent flavor and aroma. Gingerol has been extensively studied for its numerous health benefits, including its anti-inflammatory, antioxidant, and anticancer properties.

Other bioactive compounds present in ginger include shogaol, paradol, and zingerone. Shogaol, which is formed when ginger is dried or cooked, has been found to possess antioxidant, anti-inflammatory, and anticancer properties. Paradol and zingerone are lesser-known compounds, but they have also been shown to exhibit antioxidant and anti-inflammatory effects.

3.4 Antioxidants

Ginger is rich in antioxidants, which help protect the body from the damaging effects of free radicals. Free radicals are unstable molecules that can cause oxidative stress, leading to cellular damage and contributing to chronic diseases such as cancer, heart disease, and neurodegenerative disorders.

The antioxidants present in ginger include phenolic compounds, such as gingerol, as well as flavonoids, carotenoids, and other phytochemicals. These antioxidants work together to neutralize free radicals, protect cells from oxidative stress, and support overall health and well-being.

3.5 Conclusion

Ginger's nutritional profile is a testament to its incredible versatility and potency. The combination of essential vitamins, minerals, bioactive compounds, and antioxidants found in ginger make it a powerful addition to a healthy diet.

Chapter 4: The Multifaceted Health Benefits of Ginger

Ginger's unique combination of nutritional and bioactive components has long been associated with numerous health benefits. This chapter explores the multifaceted health benefits of ginger, offering insight into the various ways this powerful root can support and enhance overall well-being.

4.1 Digestive Health

Ginger has been used for centuries to treat various digestive ailments, including nausea, vomiting, indigestion, and bloating. Its carminative properties help relax the gastrointestinal muscles, relieving gas and reducing intestinal cramping. Ginger also aids in digestion by stimulating the production of digestive enzymes, which break down food and improve nutrient absorption.

Several studies have demonstrated ginger's effectiveness in alleviating pregnancy-related nausea and vomiting, as well as nausea induced by chemotherapy or surgery. Ginger's antiemetic properties are attributed to the bioactive compounds gingerol and shogaol, which help regulate the contractions of the stomach and suppress the signals responsible for inducing nausea.

4.2 Anti-Inflammatory Effects

Ginger possesses potent anti-inflammatory properties, which can help reduce inflammation and alleviate pain associated with various inflammatory conditions. The bioactive compounds gingerol and shogaol have been shown to inhibit the production of pro-inflammatory substances, such as cytokines and prostaglandins, which play a role in the inflammatory process.

Research has suggested that ginger may be beneficial in managing the symptoms of conditions such as osteoarthritis, rheumatoid arthritis, and muscle pain. Several studies have found that ginger supplementation can reduce pain and improve physical function in individuals with osteoarthritis, making it a promising natural alternative to traditional pain-relief medications.

4.3 Antioxidant Activity

The antioxidants present in ginger help protect the body from the harmful effects of free radicals, which can cause cellular damage and contribute to chronic diseases. By neutralizing free radicals, ginger's antioxidants support overall health and help reduce the risk of conditions such as heart disease, cancer, and neurodegenerative disorders.

Ginger's antioxidant properties also play a role in supporting immune function, as they help protect immune cells from oxidative stress and promote the production of immune-boosting molecules.

4.4 Cardiovascular Health

Ginger may benefit cardiovascular health by reducing several risk factors associated with heart disease. Studies have shown that ginger can lower blood pressure, reduce blood sugar levels, and improve lipid profiles by decreasing total cholesterol, triglycerides, and LDL cholesterol, while increasing HDL cholesterol.

These effects are likely due to ginger's anti-inflammatory and antioxidant properties, which help protect blood vessels from damage and prevent the formation of blood clots.

4.5 Cancer Prevention and Treatment

Emerging research has suggested that ginger may possess anticancer properties, which could help prevent and treat various types of cancer. The bioactive compounds gingerol and shogaol have been found to induce apoptosis (cell death) in cancer cells, inhibit the growth of tumors, and suppress the formation of blood vessels that supply nutrients to cancerous tissues.

While further research is needed to fully understand the mechanisms behind ginger's anticancer effects, these preliminary findings hold promise for the potential role of ginger in cancer prevention and treatment.

4.6 Diabetes Management

Ginger may help manage diabetes by improving insulin sensitivity and reducing blood sugar levels. Studies have shown that ginger supplementation can lower fasting blood sugar levels and improve long-term blood sugar control, as measured by HbA1c levels.

Additionally, ginger's antioxidant properties may help protect against the oxidative stress and inflammation associated with diabetes, further supporting overall health in individuals with this condition.

4.7 Respiratory Health

Ginger has long been used as a natural remedy for respiratory issues, such as colds, coughs, and asthma. Its anti-inflammatory and antioxidant properties help soothe irritated airways, reduce inflammation, and thin mucus, which can provide relief from congestion and coughing.

Moreover, ginger has been shown to have bronchodilatory effects, meaning it can help relax and open up the airways, making it easier to breathe. This may be particularly beneficial for individuals with asthma or other respiratory conditions.

4.8 Menstrual Pain Relief

Ginger has been found to be effective in relieving menstrual pain, also known as dysmenorrhea. Studies have shown that ginger supplementation can reduce the severity of menstrual pain, with some evidence suggesting that it may be as effective as some nonsteroidal anti-inflammatory drugs (NSAIDs) in providing relief.

The pain-relieving properties of ginger are likely due to its anti-inflammatory effects, which help reduce the production of prostaglandins, compounds responsible for the pain and inflammation associated with menstrual cramps.

4.9 Antimicrobial and Antiviral Properties

Ginger has been found to possess antimicrobial and antiviral properties, which can help protect the body against various pathogens. The bioactive compounds in ginger, such as gingerol and shogaol, have been shown to inhibit the growth of bacteria, fungi, and viruses, including some drug-resistant strains. These antimicrobial properties may help prevent and treat various infections, such as respiratory infections, foodborne illnesses, and skin infections. Additionally, ginger's antiviral effects may help support immune function and reduce the severity and duration of viral illnesses, such as the common cold and the flu.

4.10 Cognitive Function and Neuroprotection

Emerging research suggests that ginger may have potential benefits for cognitive function and neuroprotection. The antioxidants and anti-inflammatory compounds present in ginger have been shown to protect brain cells from oxidative stress and inflammation, which can contribute to neurodegenerative diseases, such as Alzheimer's disease and Parkinson's disease.

Some studies have also found that ginger supplementation can improve cognitive function and memory in both healthy individuals and those with cognitive impairments. While further research is needed to confirm these findings, ginger's potential neuroprotective effects hold promise for the prevention and treatment of cognitive decline and neurodegenerative disorders.

4.11 Conclusion

The multifaceted health benefits of ginger are a testament to the power and versatility of this remarkable root. From supporting digestive health and reducing inflammation to promoting cardiovascular health and potentially preventing cancer, ginger offers a wide range of therapeutic properties that can enhance overall well-being.

Chapter 5: Ginger and Traditional Medicine: A Global Perspective

Ginger has been used as a medicinal plant for thousands of years across various cultures and regions. This chapter explores ginger's role in traditional medicine systems around the world, providing a global perspective on the ancient wisdom and practices that have long valued ginger as a potent natural remedy.

5.1 Traditional Chinese Medicine (TCM)

In Traditional Chinese Medicine (TCM), ginger has been used for over 2,000 years to treat a variety of ailments. It is considered a warming herb, helping to balance the body's energies and restore harmony. Ginger is commonly used to treat digestive issues, such as nausea, vomiting, bloating, and diarrhea. It is also believed to help expel „wind," or excess gas, from the body.

Ginger's warming properties are thought to improve blood circulation and alleviate pain associated with conditions like arthritis and muscle aches. Additionally, ginger is used in TCM to treat respiratory issues, such as colds, coughs, and asthma, by warming the lungs and dispelling phlegm.

5.2 Ayurveda

In Ayurveda, the traditional medicine system of India, ginger is known as „vishwabheshaja," which translates to „universal medicine." It is highly valued for its various therapeutic properties, which align with the Ayurvedic principle of balancing the body's three doshas: Vata, Pitta, and Kapha.

Ginger's warming and digestive properties make it an effective remedy for balancing the Vata dosha, which is associated with coldness and movement. It is used to treat digestive issues, such as indigestion, bloating, and constipation, as well as to alleviate pain and inflammation.

Ginger is also believed to help balance the Kapha dosha, which is associated with heaviness and sluggishness. Its stimulating and expectorant properties make it an effective remedy for respiratory issues, such as colds, coughs, and sinus congestion.

5.3 Traditional Japanese Medicine (Kampo)

In traditional Japanese medicine, known as Kampo, ginger is a key ingredient in many herbal formulas. It is used to treat a wide range of conditions, including digestive issues, respiratory ailments, and circulatory disorders.

One popular Kampo remedy that includes ginger is „shoga-yu," a ginger-infused hot water drink used to relieve cold symptoms, such as chills, fever, and nasal congestion. Ginger is also a key component in „hange-shashin-to," an herbal formula used to treat gastrointestinal issues, such as diarrhea and abdominal pain.

5.4 Traditional Persian Medicine

In traditional Persian medicine, ginger has been used for centuries to treat various ailments, including digestive issues, respiratory disorders, and inflammatory conditions. It is often combined with other herbs and spices to create potent medicinal formulations.

Ginger is a key ingredient in „zofa," a traditional Persian remedy for coughs and colds, which combines ginger, cinnamon, and honey. It is also used to treat gastrointestinal issues, such as indigestion and bloating, by stimulating digestive secretions and improving nutrient absorption.

5.5 Traditional African Medicine

Ginger has a long history of use in traditional African medicine, particularly in West African countries, such as Nigeria and Ghana. It is commonly used to treat a variety of conditions, including digestive issues, respiratory ailments, and inflammatory disorders.

In traditional Nigerian medicine, ginger is used to treat stomachaches, diarrhea, and vomiting. It is also used as a natural remedy for colds, coughs, and asthma. In Ghana, ginger is used to treat conditions such as rheumatism, arthritis, and muscle pain, due to its anti-inflammatory and analgesic properties.

5.6 Conclusion

The use of ginger in traditional medicine systems around the world is a testament to its powerful therapeutic properties and enduring significance. From Traditional Chinese Medicine and Ayurveda to Kampo, traditional Persian medicine, and African healing practices, ginger has been valued for centuries as a potent natural remedy for a wide range of ailments.

By understanding the global perspectives and ancient wisdom that have long recognized ginger's healing potential, we can better appreciate its role in modern medicine and holistic health practices. As research continues to uncover new applications for ginger, it is important to remember the rich cultural and historical contexts that have shaped our understanding of this remarkable root.

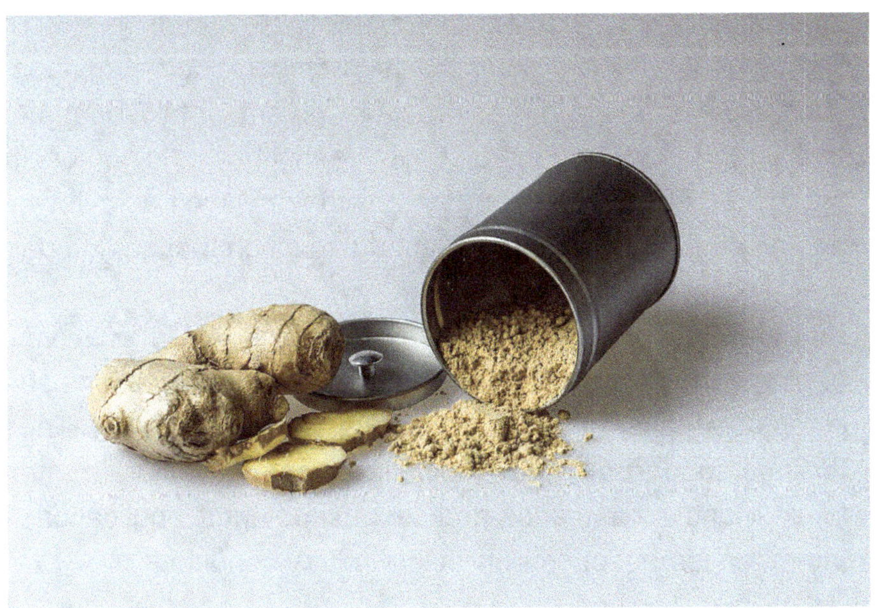

Chapter 6: Ginger in Modern Medicine: Scientific Breakthroughs

In recent years, modern scientific research has begun to uncover the underlying mechanisms behind ginger's therapeutic properties, validating its traditional uses and revealing new potential applications. This chapter explores some of the most significant scientific breakthroughs in our understanding of ginger and its role in modern medicine.

6.1 Anti-Inflammatory and Analgesic Properties

One of the most widely studied aspects of ginger is its anti-inflammatory and analgesic properties. Research has identified several bioactive compounds in ginger, such as gingerol, shogaol, and zingerone, that have potent anti-inflammatory effects. These compounds have been shown to inhibit the production of pro-inflammatory substances, such as cytokines and prostaglandins, which contribute to inflammation and pain.

Numerous clinical trials have demonstrated the effectiveness of ginger in reducing pain and inflammation in conditions such as osteoarthritis, rheumatoid arthritis, and muscle pain. These findings support ginger's traditional uses as a natural remedy for pain and inflammation and suggest potential applications in the management of chronic inflammatory conditions.

6.2 Digestive Health

Ginger's role in supporting digestive health has long been recognized in traditional medicine, and modern research has provided scientific evidence to support these claims. Studies have shown that ginger can help alleviate nausea and vomiting associated with pregnancy, chemotherapy, and surgery by acting on the gastrointestinal tract and the central nervous system.

Ginger has also been found to promote the secretion of digestive enzymes, which can help improve digestion and nutrient absorption. These findings validate ginger's traditional use as a digestive aid and highlight its potential for treating a variety of gastrointestinal issues.

6.3 Cardiovascular Health

Emerging research has revealed that ginger may have a positive impact on cardiovascular health by targeting several risk factors associated with heart disease. Studies have shown that ginger can help lower blood pressure, improve lipid profiles, and reduce blood sugar levels.

These effects are likely due to ginger's anti-inflammatory and antioxidant properties, which protect blood vessels from damage and prevent the formation of blood clots. These findings suggest that ginger may have a role to play in the prevention and management of cardiovascular disease.

6.4 Anticancer Properties

Preliminary research has suggested that ginger may possess anticancer properties, with several studies identifying bioactive compounds, such as gingerol and shogaol, that can inhibit the growth of cancer cells and induce apoptosis (cell death). Ginger's anticancer effects have been observed in various types of cancer, including breast, ovarian, pancreatic, and colorectal cancer.

While further research is needed to fully understand the mechanisms behind ginger's anticancer properties and to establish its potential role in cancer prevention and treatment, these initial findings hold promise for the development of new therapeutic strategies.

6.5 Neuroprotective Effects

Recent research has also suggested that ginger may have potential neuroprotective effects, with studies demonstrating its ability to protect brain cells from oxidative stress and inflammation. These findings suggest that ginger may have a role to play in the prevention and treatment of neurodegenerative diseases, such as Alzheimer's and Parkinson's disease.

Ginger's antioxidant and anti-inflammatory properties may also help improve cognitive function and memory, with some studies showing positive effects in both healthy individuals and those with cognitive impairments.

6.6 Conclusion

Modern scientific research has provided valuable insights into the therapeutic properties of ginger, validating many of its traditional uses and uncovering new potential applications. From its well-established anti-inflammatory and digestive benefits to its emerging roles in cardiovascular health, cancer prevention, and neuroprotection, ginger's versatility and potency make it a valuable addition to modern medicine and integrative health practices.

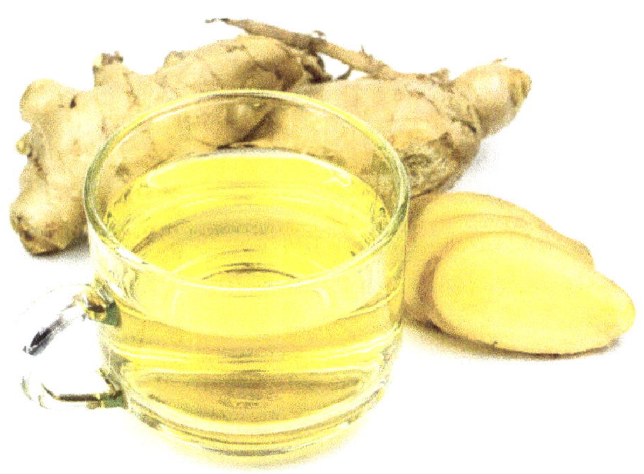

Chapter 7: Ginger Essential Oil: Extraction, Benefits, and Uses

Ginger essential oil is another way to harness the power of this versatile root. Extracted from the rhizome of the ginger plant, this concentrated oil offers many of the same health benefits as the whole root, while also providing unique applications in aromatherapy, massage, and personal care products. In this chapter, we will explore the extraction process, benefits, and uses of ginger essential oil.

7.1 Extraction of Ginger Essential Oil

Ginger essential oil is typically extracted using steam distillation, a process that involves passing steam through the crushed or ground ginger rhizomes. The steam helps release the volatile compounds, including the essential oil, which is then collected and separated from the water. This method preserves the integrity of the bioactive compounds in ginger, resulting in a pure, concentrated oil that retains its therapeutic properties.

7.2 Benefits of Ginger Essential Oil

Ginger essential oil shares many of the same benefits as the whole ginger root, thanks to its rich content of bioactive compounds, such as gingerol and zingerone. Some of the key benefits of ginger essential oil include:

- *Anti-inflammatory and analgesic effects:* Ginger essential oil can help reduce inflammation and alleviate pain, making it a popular choice for massage oils and topical treatments for conditions like arthritis, muscle aches, and joint pain.
- *Digestive support:* The warming and carminative properties of ginger essential oil can help soothe the digestive system, alleviating symptoms like nausea, indigestion, and bloating.
- *Respiratory relief:* Ginger essential oil can help clear congestion, reduce coughing, and soothe irritated airways, making it a useful addition to aromatherapy blends and inhalation treatments for respiratory issues.
- *Antimicrobial and antiviral properties:* Ginger essential oil has been found to possess antimicrobial and antiviral properties, which can help protect against infections and support immune function.
- *Mood enhancement:* The warm, spicy scent of ginger essential oil is thought to have uplifting and energizing effects, making it a popular choice for aromatherapy blends aimed at boosting mood and reducing stress.

7.3 Uses of Ginger Essential Oil

Ginger essential oil can be used in various ways to harness its therapeutic properties. Some common uses include:

- *Aromatherapy:* Diffusing ginger essential oil or incorporating it into aromatherapy blends can help support respiratory health, boost mood, and promote relaxation. Combining ginger essential oil with complementary oils, such as lemon, orange, or eucalyptus, can enhance its therapeutic effects.

- *Massage oil:* Diluting ginger essential oil in a carrier oil, such as almond or jojoba oil, creates a warming massage oil that can help relieve muscle and joint pain, as well as improve circulation.
- *Topical applications:* Ginger essential oil can be added to creams, lotions, and salves for topical treatments targeting inflammation, pain, and skin issues. Always dilute the essential oil in a carrier oil or cream before applying it to the skin to avoid irritation.
- *Inhalation:* Inhaling ginger essential oil, either directly from the bottle or by adding a few drops to a bowl of hot water, can help clear nasal congestion and soothe respiratory symptoms.
- *Personal care products:* Ginger essential oil can be added to homemade soaps, shampoos, and bath products, providing a warm, invigorating scent and potential health benefits.

7.4 Conclusion

Ginger essential oil is a versatile and potent way to experience the many benefits of ginger. From its anti-inflammatory and digestive properties to its uplifting scent, ginger essential oil offers a range of applications in aromatherapy, massage, and personal care.

Chapter 8: Ginger in the Culinary World: Flavor, Spice, and Versatility

Ginger has long been valued not only for its medicinal properties but also for its unique and versatile flavor profile. Used in a wide range of cuisines, ginger brings warmth, spiciness, and a subtle sweetness to both savory and sweet dishes. In this chapter, we will explore the use of ginger in the culinary world, examining its many applications and offering tips on how to incorporate this powerful spice into your own cooking.

8.1 Flavor Profile of Ginger

Ginger has a distinct flavor profile that can be described as warm, spicy, and slightly sweet with a hint of citrus. Its pungent and aromatic qualities make it a popular ingredient in many cuisines around the world, particularly in Asian, Indian, and Caribbean cooking. In addition to its fresh, zesty taste, ginger also has a unique texture, with fibrous, juicy flesh that can be grated, minced, or sliced for various culinary applications.

8.2 Fresh Ginger vs. Dried Ginger

Ginger is available in various forms, including fresh, dried, and powdered. Fresh ginger, with its juicy and aromatic qualities, is often preferred for its more potent flavor and versatility. Dried ginger, which can be found as whole pieces or ground into a powder, has a more concentrated flavor and a longer shelf life, making it a convenient option for those who don't have access to fresh ginger or need it for specific recipes.

While fresh and dried ginger can often be used interchangeably in recipes, it's essential to adjust the quantities accordingly, as dried ginger has a more intense flavor. A general rule of thumb is to use about one-third the amount of dried ginger as you would fresh ginger.

8.3 Culinary Applications of Ginger

Ginger's unique flavor profile lends itself to a wide range of culinary applications, from savory dishes and beverages to sweet treats and desserts. Some popular uses for ginger in cooking include:

- *Stir-fries:* Ginger is a staple ingredient in many Asian stir-fries, where it is often combined with garlic, soy sauce, and other flavorful ingredients to create a rich and aromatic sauce.
- *Curries:* In Indian cuisine, ginger is frequently used in curry dishes, imparting warmth and depth to the complex spice blends that characterize these flavorful stews.
- *Marinades and dressings:* Ginger can be used in marinades and dressings for meat, fish, and vegetables, adding a burst of flavor and tenderizing the protein.
- *Soups and stews:* Ginger's warming and soothing qualities make it a popular addition to soups and stews, particularly in Asian and Caribbean cuisines.

- *Baking:* Ground ginger is a common ingredient in baked goods, such as gingerbread cookies, ginger snaps, and spiced cakes. Its warm, sweet flavor pairs well with other spices like cinnamon, nutmeg, and cloves.
- *Beverages:* Ginger can be used to flavor a variety of beverages, from soothing teas and invigorating smoothies to spicy cocktails and mocktails.

8.4 Tips for Cooking with Ginger

When cooking with ginger, keep the following tips in mind to make the most of its unique flavor and health benefits:

- Store fresh ginger in a cool, dark place or in the refrigerator to prolong its freshness.
- To easily peel fresh ginger, use the edge of a spoon to scrape away the thin skin.
- Grate, mince, or slice fresh ginger to release its aromatic oils and maximize its flavor.
- When using dried ginger, store it in an airtight container away from heat and light to preserve its potency.
- Experiment with different forms of ginger (fresh, dried, pickled, or crystallized) to find the flavor and texture that best suit your recipes
- Try combining ginger with other spices and flavors, such as garlic, soy sauce, lime, or honey, to create well-rounded and harmonious taste profiles.
- Remember that ginger's flavor can intensify as it cooks, so it's a good idea to start with a small amount and adjust to taste as needed.

- To mellow out ginger's spiciness, try sautéing or roasting it before adding it to a dish. This will also help to release its aromatic oils and enhance its flavor.

8.5 Ginger in Traditional and Fusion Cuisine

Ginger's versatility and distinctive flavor have made it a popular ingredient in traditional dishes from various cultures. Here are some examples of how ginger is used in traditional and fusion cuisines:

- *Chinese cuisine:* Ginger is a fundamental ingredient in many Chinese dishes, such as ginger and scallion chicken, ginger beef, and ginger garlic shrimp. It is often paired with garlic and green onions for a balanced and aromatic flavor profile.
- *Indian cuisine:* Ginger plays a central role in Indian cooking, featuring prominently in curry dishes, chutneys, and spice blends like garam masala. It is also used in Indian sweets like ginger-infused rice pudding and ginger-spiced tea.
- *Japanese cuisine:* Ginger is commonly used in Japanese cooking, both in its fresh and pickled forms. Pickled ginger, or gari, is often served alongside sushi as a palate cleanser, while fresh ginger can be found in dishes like teriyaki and tempura.
- *Caribbean cuisine:* In Caribbean cooking, ginger is frequently used in marinades, sauces, and spice blends. Dishes like Jamaican jerk chicken and Trinidadian curry often feature ginger as a key flavor component.

- *Fusion cuisine:* As chefs continue to experiment with bold and creative flavor combinations, ginger has found its way into various fusion dishes. For example, ginger-infused chocolate truffles, ginger lime ceviche, and ginger-glazed salmon all showcase the root's adaptability and flair in contemporary cooking.

8.6 Conclusion

Ginger's unique and versatile flavor profile makes it a valuable addition to any kitchen. From traditional Asian, Indian, and Caribbean dishes to innovative fusion creations, ginger's warmth, spiciness, and subtle sweetness can elevate a wide variety of recipes. By understanding its culinary applications and experimenting with different forms and flavor pairings, you can unlock the full potential of this powerful spice in your own cooking

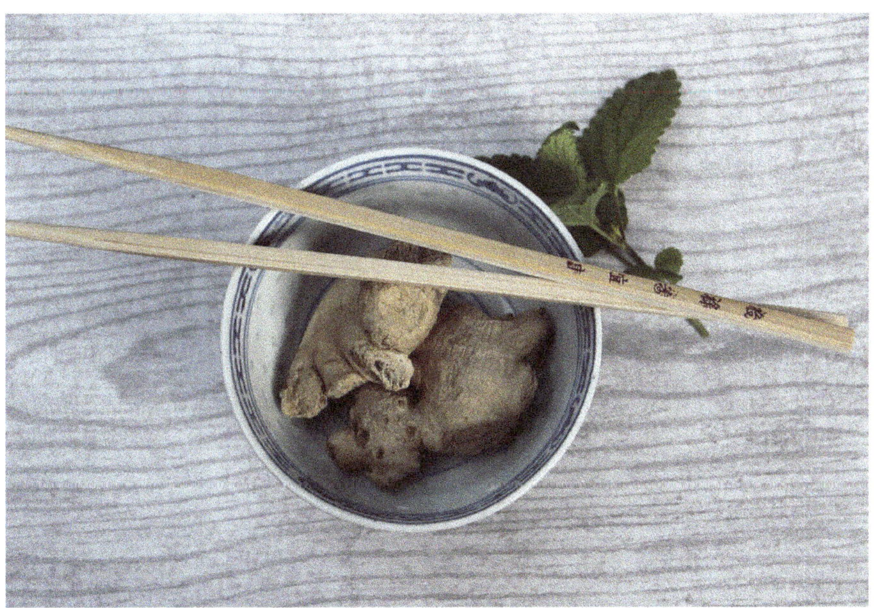

Chapter 9: Innovative Ginger Recipes: From Appetizers to Desserts

With its unique flavor profile and numerous health benefits, ginger is a versatile ingredient that can be incorporated into a wide variety of dishes. In this chapter, we will explore innovative ginger recipes that showcase the root's potential in every course of a meal, from appetizers and main dishes to beverages and desserts.

9.1 Ginger-Spiced Hummus

This twist on classic hummus adds warmth and depth to the creamy chickpea dip with the addition of ginger, making it perfect for a flavorful appetizer or snack.

Ingredients:

1 15-ounce can chickpeas, drained and rinsed
1/4 cup tahini
3 tablespoons lemon juice
2 tablespoons extra-virgin olive oil
2 cloves garlic, minced
1-inch piece fresh ginger, peeled and grated
1/2 teaspoon ground cumin
1/2 teaspoon paprika
Salt and pepper, to taste

Instructions:

In a food processor, combine the chickpeas, tahini, lemon juice, olive oil, garlic, ginger, cumin, and paprika. Process until smooth, scraping down the sides as needed.
Season the hummus with salt and pepper to taste, adjusting the flavors as desired.
Serve the ginger-spiced hummus with pita bread, fresh vegetables, or crackers for dipping.

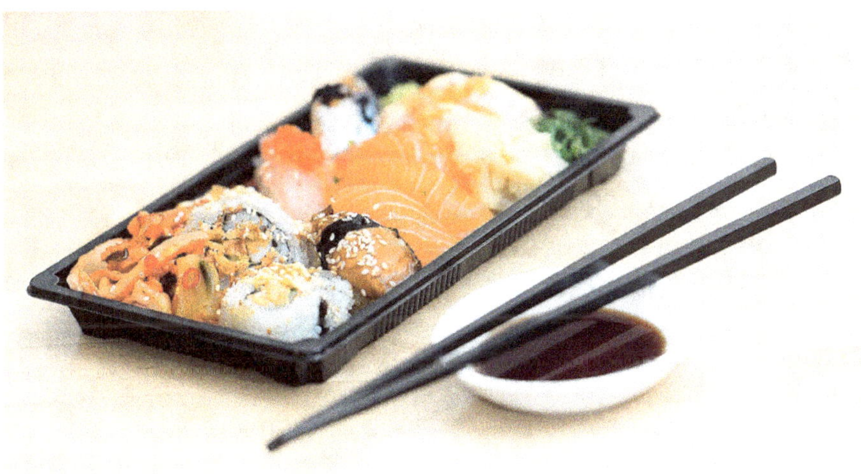

9.2 Ginger Coconut Curry

This fragrant and flavorful curry, infused with ginger and coconut milk, is an excellent way to showcase ginger's potential in savory dishes.

Ingredients:

2 tablespoons coconut oil
1 onion, diced
1 red bell pepper, sliced
2 cloves garlic, minced
1-inch piece fresh ginger, minced
1 tablespoon curry powder
1 teaspoon ground turmeric
1 teaspoon ground coriander
1 14-ounce can coconut milk
1 14-ounce can diced tomatoes
4 cups assorted vegetables (such as cauliflower, carrots, and green beans)
1 15-ounce can chickpeas, drained and rinsed
Salt and pepper, to taste
Fresh cilantro, for garnish

Instructions:

In a large pot or Dutch oven, heat the coconut oil over medium heat. Add the onion and bell pepper and cook until softened, about 5 minutes.

Stir in the garlic, ginger, curry powder, turmeric, and coriander, and cook for another minute, until fragrant.

Add the coconut milk, diced tomatoes, vegetables, and chickpeas, stirring to combine. Bring the mixture to a simmer, then reduce the heat and cook, covered, for 20-25 minutes, until the vegetables are tender.

Season the curry with salt and pepper to taste. Serve over rice or with flatbread, garnished with fresh cilantro.

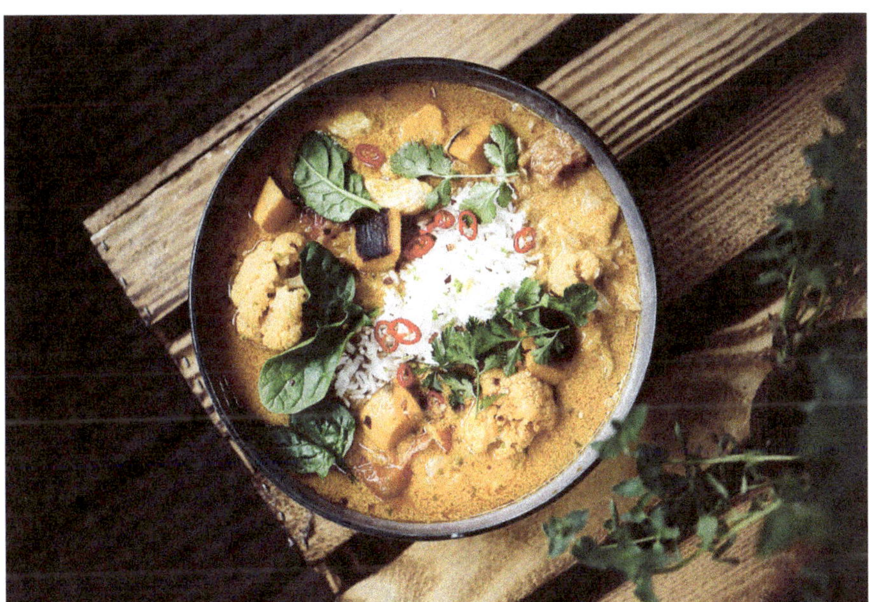

9.3 Ginger Mango Smoothie

This refreshing and invigorating smoothie, featuring ginger, mango, and a hint of lime, is perfect for a morning boost or an afternoon pick-me-up.

Ingredients:

1 cup frozen mango chunks
1/2 banana, peeled
1/2 cup unsweetened almond milk
1/4 cup Greek yogurt
1 tablespoon honey or maple syrup
1-inch piece fresh ginger, peeled and grated
1 tablespoon lime juice
1/2 cup ice

Instructions:

In a blender, combine the mango, banana, almond milk, Greek yogurt, honey or maple syrup, ginger, lime juice, and ice.
Blend until smooth and creamy, adjusting the consistency with more almond milk or ice as needed.
Pour the smoothie into a glass and enjoy immediately for the best taste and texture.

9.4 Ginger Soy Glazed Salmon

This simple yet flavorful ginger soy glazed salmon is a delicious way to incorporate ginger into your main course, with a balance of sweet, savory, and spicy flavors.

Ingredients:

4 salmon fillets, skin-on
1/4 cup soy sauce
1/4 cup honey
2 tablespoons rice vinegar
2 cloves garlic, minced
1-inch piece fresh ginger, peeled and minced
1 tablespoon sesame oil
2 green onions, thinly sliced
1 tablespoon sesame seeds

Instructions:

Preheat your oven to 400°F (200°C).
In a small saucepan, combine the soy sauce, honey, rice vinegar, garlic, and ginger. Bring the mixture to a simmer over medium heat, and cook until slightly thickened, about 5 minutes.

Place the salmon fillets on a foil-lined baking sheet and brush with the sesame oil. Spoon the ginger soy glaze over the salmon, reserving some for serving.

Bake the salmon for 12-15 minutes, or until cooked to your desired level of doneness.

Remove the salmon from the oven and let rest for a few minutes before serving. Drizzle with the reserved ginger soy glaze and garnish with sliced green onions and sesame seeds.

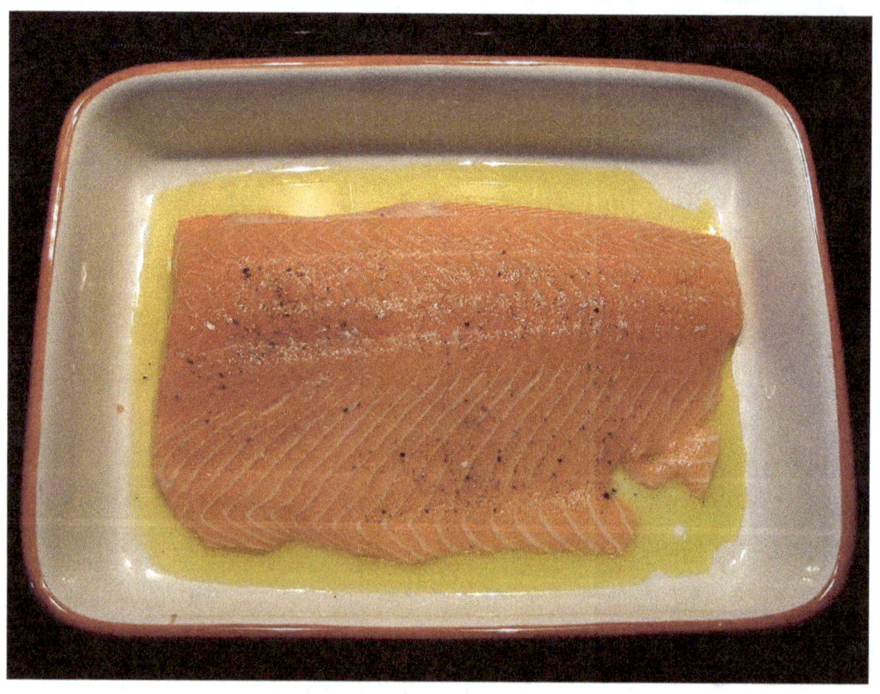

9.5 Ginger Pear Crisp

This ginger pear crisp combines the natural sweetness of ripe pears with the warmth of ginger and cinnamon, making it a delightful and comforting dessert.

Ingredients:

4 ripe pears, peeled, cored, and sliced
2 tablespoons lemon juice
1/4 cup granulated sugar
1 tablespoon cornstarch
1 teaspoon ground ginger
1/2 teaspoon ground cinnamon

Topping:

1 cup old-fashioned rolled oats
1/2 cup all-purpose flour
1/2 cup brown sugar
1/2 teaspoon ground ginger
1/4 teaspoon ground cinnamon
1/4 teaspoon salt
6 tablespoons unsalted butter, cut into small pieces

Instructions:

- Preheat your oven to 350°F (175°C). Grease an 8-inch square baking dish.

- In a large bowl, combine the sliced pears, lemon juice, granulated sugar, cornstarch, ginger, and cinnamon. Mix well to coat the pears evenly, then transfer the mixture to the prepared baking dish.

- In another bowl, combine the oats, flour, brown sugar, ginger, cinnamon, and salt. Using your fingers or a pastry cutter, cut in the butter until the mixture resembles coarse crumbs.

- Sprinkle the topping evenly over the pear mixture in the baking dish.

- Bake the ginger pear crisp for 35-45 minutes, or until the topping is golden brown and the pears are bubbling and tender.
- Remove the crisp from the oven and let cool slightly before serving. Enjoy warm, with a scoop of vanilla ice cream or a dollop of whipped cream, if desired.

These innovative ginger recipes showcase the versatility and unique flavor profile of this powerful root, inspiring you to incorporate it into a wide range of dishes, from appetizers and main courses to beverages and desserts. As you continue to explore the world of ginger, you'll discover countless ways to enjoy its many benefits and delicious taste.

Chapter 10: Ginger Beverages: Teas, Tonics, and Cocktails

Ginger's distinctive flavor and health benefits make it an excellent addition to a variety of beverages. In this chapter, we will explore different ways to incorporate ginger into teas, tonics, and cocktails, offering refreshing and invigorating options for any occasion.

10.1 Ginger Tea

Ginger tea is a popular and soothing beverage with numerous health benefits, including digestive support and anti-inflammatory properties.

Ingredients:

1-inch piece fresh ginger, peeled and thinly sliced
2 cups water
1 tablespoon honey or sweetener of choice (optional)
1 tablespoon lemon juice (optional)

Instructions:

- In a small saucepan, combine the ginger slices and water. Bring the mixture to a boil, then reduce the heat and simmer for 10-15 minutes.

- Strain the tea into a cup, discarding the ginger slices. If desired, add honey or your preferred sweetener and lemon juice to taste.

- Enjoy the ginger tea hot or let it cool and serve over ice for a refreshing iced ginger tea.

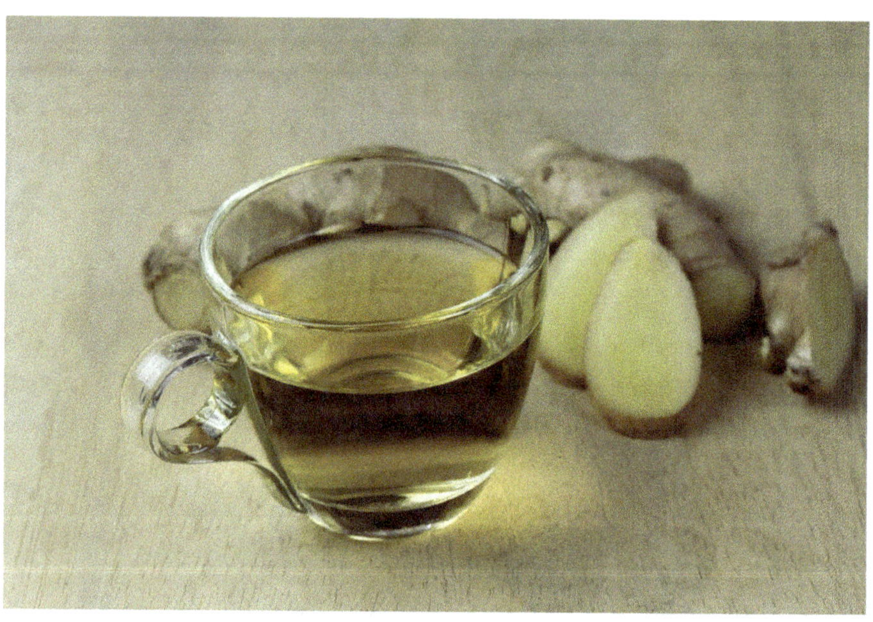

10.2 Ginger Turmeric Tonic

This ginger turmeric tonic is a nutrient-rich and invigorating beverage, perfect for boosting immunity and supporting overall health.

Ingredients:

1-inch piece fresh ginger, peeled and chopped
1-inch piece fresh turmeric, peeled and chopped (or 1 teaspoon ground turmeric)
2 cups coconut water
1/2 cup fresh orange juice
2 tablespoons lemon juice
1 tablespoon honey or sweetener of choice
Pinch of black pepper

Instructions:

- In a blender, combine the ginger, turmeric, coconut water, orange juice, lemon juice, honey or sweetener, and black pepper. Blend until smooth.
- Strain the mixture through a fine-mesh sieve or nut milk bag to remove any solids.
- Serve the ginger turmeric tonic over ice or chill in the refrigerator before enjoying.

10.3 Ginger Beer

Ginger beer is a non-alcoholic, fermented beverage that is both sweet and spicy, making it a delicious and refreshing drink on its own or as a mixer in cocktails.

Ingredients:

1/4 cup grated fresh ginger
1/4 cup granulated sugar
1/4 cup fresh lemon juice
1/4 teaspoon active dry yeast
4 cups filtered water

Instructions:

- In a clean, sterilized 2-liter plastic bottle, combine the ginger, sugar, lemon juice, and yeast. Add the filtered water, leaving about 1 inch of headspace at the top of the bottle.
- Secure the cap tightly and shake the bottle to dissolve the sugar and distribute the yeast. Let the bottle sit at room temperature for 24-48 hours, occasionally releasing the pressure by slightly unscrewing the cap.
- When the ginger beer has become carbonated, strain it through a fine-mesh sieve or cheesecloth to remove the ginger solids. Transfer the ginger beer to a clean bottle or container and refrigerate to chill.
- Enjoy the ginger beer on its own, or use it as a mixer in cocktails like a Moscow Mule or Dark and Stormy.

10.4 Ginger Basil Smash Cocktail

This ginger basil smash cocktail is a refreshing and sophisticated drink, combining the flavors of ginger, basil, and lemon for a unique and delightful libation.

Ingredients:

2 ounces gin
1/2 ounce fresh lemon juice
1/2 ounce simple syrup
1-inch piece fresh ginger, peeled and thinly sliced
6-8 fresh basil leaves
Ice
Sodawater, for topping (optional)

Instructions:

- In a cocktail shaker, muddle the ginger slices and basil leaves to release their flavors.
- Add the gin, lemon juice, simple syrup, and a handful of ice to the shaker. Shake vigorously for about 15 seconds to chill and combine the ingredients.
- Strain the cocktail into a glass filled with fresh ice. If desired, top with a splash of soda water for a bit of effervescence.
- Garnish with a sprig of basil or a lemon twist, and enjoy your ginger basil smash cocktail.

10.5 Ginger Hot Toddy

A ginger hot toddy is a comforting and warming beverage, perfect for sipping on chilly evenings or when you're feeling under the weather.

Ingredients:

1 1/2 ounces whiskey or bourbon
1 tablespoon honey or sweetener of choice
1-inch piece fresh ginger, peeled and thinly sliced
1/2 lemon, juiced
1 cinnamon stick
Boiling water

Instructions:

- In a heatproof glass or mug, combine the whiskey or bourbon, honey or sweetener, ginger slices, and lemon juice.
- Top with boiling water, filling the glass or mug to your desired level.
- Stir gently with a cinnamon stick, allowing it to steep in the hot toddy for a minute or two before removing.
- Sip the ginger hot toddy while it's still warm, enjoying the soothing and warming effects of the ginger, lemon, and cinnamon.

- In this chapter, we have explored various ways to incorporate ginger into your beverages, from soothing teas and nutrient-rich tonics to refreshing cocktails. The versatility and unique flavor of ginger make it a wonderful addition to your drink repertoire, providing both delicious taste and numerous health benefits.

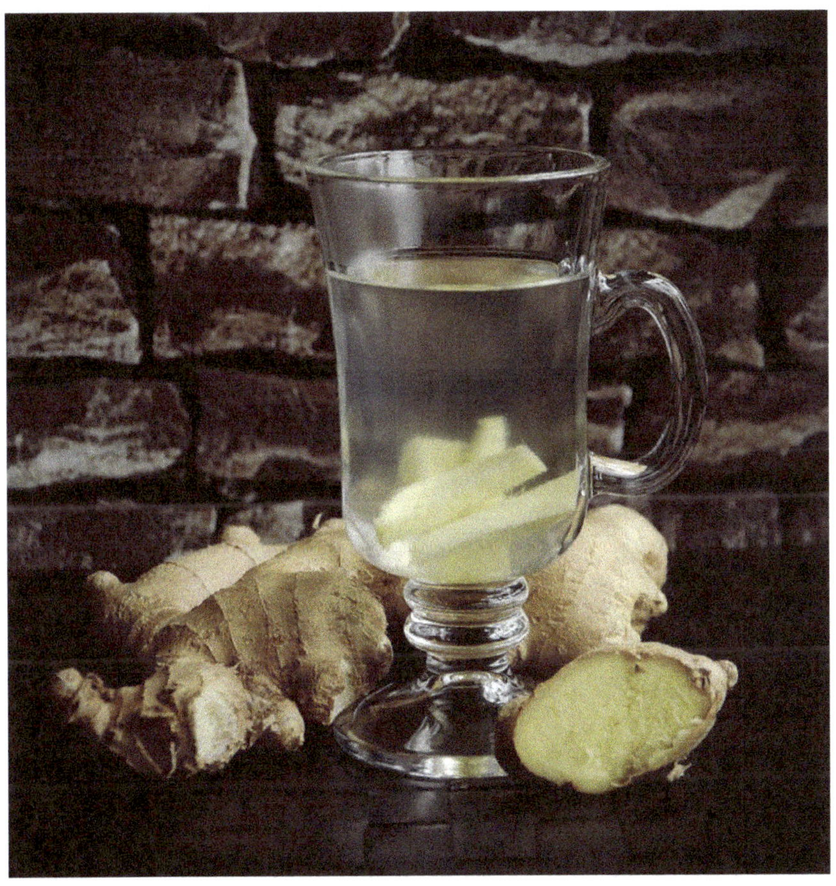

Chapter 11: Ginger in Skincare and Beauty: Natural Remedies and Treatments

Ginger's natural properties, such as antioxidants and anti-inflammatory compounds, make it an excellent ingredient for skincare and beauty treatments. In this chapter, we will explore ways to harness the benefits of ginger for your skin, hair, and overall well-being.

11.1 Ginger Face Mask for Glowing Skin

This simple ginger face mask can help brighten your complexion and reduce inflammation, leaving your skin with a healthy glow.

Ingredients:

1 teaspoon grated fresh ginger
1 tablespoon honey
1 tablespoon plain yogurt

Instructions:

- In a small bowl, combine the grated ginger, honey, and yogurt. Mix well to form a smooth paste.

- Apply the ginger face mask to clean, dry skin, avoiding the eye area. Leave the mask on for 10-15 minutes.
- Rinse off the mask with lukewarm water, gently massaging your skin in circular motions as you remove the mask.
- Pat your skin dry and follow up with your regular skincare routine.

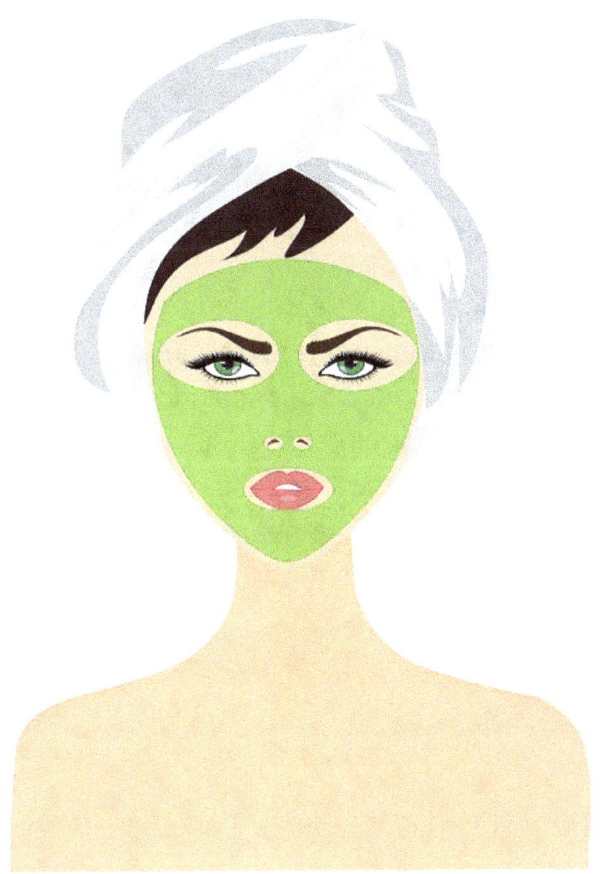

11.2 Ginger Scalp Treatment for Hair Growth

Ginger's anti-inflammatory properties can help stimulate hair growth and soothe an irritated scalp.

Ingredients:

1 tablespoon grated fresh ginger
2 tablespoons coconut oil or jojoba oil

Instructions:

- In a small bowl, mix the grated ginger with the oil of your choice.
- Apply the ginger scalp treatment to your scalp, massaging it in with your fingertips for a few minutes.
- Leave the treatment on your scalp for at least 30 minutes, or overnight for more intense results.
- Wash your hair with your regular shampoo, making sure to thoroughly remove the ginger and oil mixture.
- Use this treatment once or twice a week to promote hair growth and a healthy scalp.

11.3 Ginger Bath Soak for Relaxation and Muscle Relief

A ginger bath soak can help ease sore muscles, reduce inflammation, and promote relaxation.

Ingredients:

1/2 cup grated fresh ginger
1/2 cup Epsom salt
5-10 drops essential oil of choice (optional)

Instructions:

- Fill your bathtub with warm water.
- In a small bowl, mix the grated ginger, Epsom salt, and essential oil if using. Stir well to combine.
- Add the ginger bath soak mixture to the running bathwater, allowing it to dissolve and disperse throughout the tub.
- Soak in the ginger-infused bath for 20-30 minutes, enjoying the soothing and warming effects of the ginger.
- Rinse off your body with fresh water after your bath, and pat yourself dry with a clean towel.

11.4 Ginger Lip Scrub for Soft, Smooth Lips

This ginger lip scrub gently exfoliates and nourishes your lips, leaving them soft and smooth.

Ingredients:

1 teaspoon grated fresh ginger
1 tablespoon brown sugar
1 tablespoon coconut oil or olive oil

Instructions:

- In a small bowl, mix the grated ginger, brown sugar, and oil of your choice. Stir well to combine.
- Apply a small amount of the ginger lip scrub to your lips, gently massaging it in with your fingertips or a soft toothbrush.
- Rinse off the lip scrub with lukewarm water, and pat your lips dry with a clean towel.
- Follow up with a nourishing lip balm to keep your lips moisturized.
- These natural ginger remedies and treatments showcase the versatility of this powerful root in skincare and beauty applications. By incorporating ginger into your self-care routine, you can harness its numerous benefits for your skin, hair, and overall well-being.

Chapter 12: Growing Ginger at Home: From Seed to Harvest

Growing ginger at home is an exciting and rewarding endeavor. Not only will you have a steady supply of fresh ginger to use in cooking, skincare, and natural remedies, but you'll also gain a deeper appreciation for this versatile plant. In this chapter, we will guide you through the process of growing ginger at home, from seed to harvest.

12.1 Selecting Ginger Rhizomes

To grow ginger at home, you'll need to start with a healthy ginger rhizome (the underground stem). Look for plump, fresh ginger rhizomes with multiple „eyes" or growth buds, similar to those found on a potato. You can purchase ginger rhizomes from a local nursery or garden center, or use store-bought ginger as long as it is fresh and organic.

12.2 Preparing the Ginger Rhizomes

Before planting, soak the ginger rhizomes in warm water for several hours or overnight to help stimulate growth. You can also cut the rhizome into smaller pieces, each with at least one eye or growth bud, to produce multiple ginger plants. Allow the cut surfaces to dry and form a callus for a day or two before planting.

12.3 Planting Ginger

Ginger thrives in well-draining, fertile soil with a pH of 6.0-6.5. You can grow ginger in the ground if you live in a region with a warm, tropical climate, or in containers if you live in a cooler climate. Plant the ginger rhizomes 1-2 inches deep, with the growth buds facing upward. Space the rhizomes about 12 inches apart to give them room to grow.

12.4 Caring for Your Ginger Plants

Ginger plants require the following care to grow successfully:

- *Light:* Ginger prefers partial shade or dappled sunlight. If growing ginger in containers, place them in a spot that receives morning sun and afternoon shade.
- *Water:* Keep the soil consistently moist but not waterlogged. Ginger plants need regular watering, especially during hot or dry weather.
- *Fertilizer:* Feed your ginger plants with a balanced, slow-release fertilizer or organic compost every 4-6 weeks during the growing season.

12.5 Overwintering Ginger

If you live in a region with cold winters, you'll need to overwinter your ginger plants indoors. Bring container-grown ginger plants indoors before the first frost, placing them in a sunny, well-ventilated spot. Reduce watering and allow the foliage to die back naturally. In late winter, resume regular watering to encourage new growth.

12.6 Harvesting Ginger

Ginger takes about 8-10 months to reach maturity, depending on the growing conditions. You can harvest young ginger, with a milder flavor and thin skin, after 4-6 months. Mature ginger, with a stronger flavor and thicker skin, can be harvested when the leaves start to yellow and die back.

To harvest ginger, carefully dig around the base of the plant, lifting the rhizome with a garden fork or your hands. Break off the amount of ginger you need, leaving the rest of the rhizome in the ground to continue growing. Rinse the harvested ginger and allow it to air-dry before storing or using.

In this chapter, we have explored the process of growing ginger at home, from selecting and preparing ginger rhizomes to planting, caring for, and harvesting your ginger plants. By growing your own ginger, you'll have a fresh and abundant supply to use in various ways, while also enjoying the satisfaction of cultivating this versatile and valuable plant.

Chapter 13: The Global Ginger Trade: Economics, Sustainability, and Fair Practices

Ginger, a prized spice and medicinal plant, has a long history of cultivation and trade around the world. As demand for ginger continues to grow, it's important to understand the economics, sustainability, and fair practices involved in the global ginger trade. In this chapter, we'll explore these aspects and their impact on farmers, consumers, and the environment.

13.1 The Economics of Ginger

Ginger is a high-value crop with a global market. The main ginger-producing countries include India, China, Nigeria, Indonesia, and Nepal, while the top importers are the United States, Japan, and various European countries. Ginger is traded in various forms, including fresh, dried, powdered, and processed into essential oils and other products.

As the demand for ginger grows, driven by its culinary, medicinal, and cosmetic uses, the market is expected to expand. This presents opportunities for ginger farmers to improve their livelihoods, but it also leads to increased competition and potential price fluctuations.

13.2 Sustainability in Ginger Production

Sustainable ginger production is essential for preserving natural resources, minimizing environmental impact, and ensuring long-term viability for farmers. Key aspects of sustainable ginger farming include:

- *Organic farming practices:* Using natural pest control methods, composting, and crop rotation to maintain soil fertility and reduce the reliance on synthetic chemicals.
- *Water conservation:* Employing efficient irrigation techniques and rainwater harvesting to minimize water usage.
- *Soil conservation:* Implementing practices such as contour farming and terracing to prevent soil erosion and maintain soil health.

Supporting sustainable ginger production can help protect the environment, ensure a stable supply of ginger, and promote healthier products for consumers.

13.3 Fair Trade and Ethical Practices

Fair trade practices aim to ensure that farmers receive a fair price for their ginger, enabling them to improve their living conditions, invest in their farms, and contribute to their communities. Ethical practices in the ginger trade also encompass workers' rights, such as fair wages, safe working conditions, and the prohibition of child labor.

Certification programs, such as Fair Trade and Rainforest Alliance, help promote fair and ethical practices in the ginger trade by setting standards and providing a recognizable label for consumers. By choosing certified ginger products, consumers can support farmers and contribute to the development of more equitable and sustainable trade practices.

13.4 Challenges and Opportunities in the Ginger Trade

While the global ginger trade presents opportunities for economic growth and development, it also faces several challenges, including:

- *Climate change:* Changes in temperature and rainfall patterns can affect ginger yields, making it difficult for farmers to maintain a stable income.
- *Pests and diseases:* Ginger crops are susceptible to various pests and diseases, which can lead to significant losses if not properly managed.
- *Market fluctuations:* Changes in global demand, competition, and trade policies can impact ginger prices and make it challenging for farmers to plan for the future.

Addressing these challenges requires collaborative efforts among farmers, industry stakeholders, governments, and consumers to develop resilient and sustainable ginger production systems and support fair trade practices.

In this chapter, we have examined the global ginger trade's economics, sustainability, and fair practices. By understanding the complex interplay of these factors, we can make informed choices as consumers and support the development of a more equitable and environmentally responsible ginger industry.

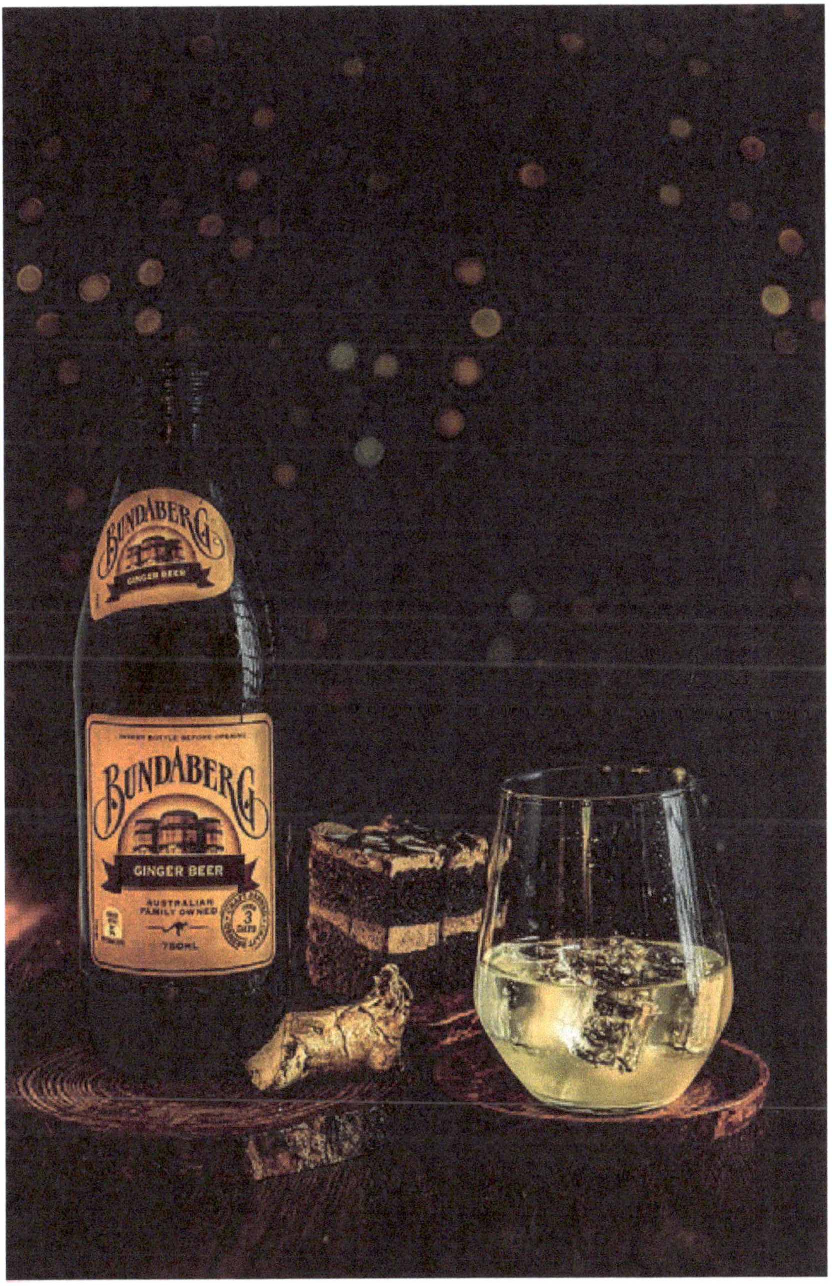

Chapter 14: The Future of Ginger: Research, Innovations, and Potential Applications

As interest in ginger continues to grow, researchers and innovators are exploring new ways to utilize this versatile plant's properties. In this chapter, we'll examine ongoing research, innovations, and potential applications for ginger in various fields, from medicine and agriculture to technology and sustainability.

14.1 Ginger in Medicine and Healthcare

Ginger's potential health benefits have been the subject of numerous studies, and researchers continue to investigate its properties and applications. Future areas of interest include:

- *Cancer treatment:* Some studies suggest that ginger's bioactive compounds may have anti-cancer properties, such as inhibiting tumor growth and inducing cell death in cancer cells. Further research is needed to confirm these findings and explore ginger's potential role in cancer prevention and treatment.
- *Diabetes management:* Preliminary research indicates that ginger may help regulate blood sugar levels and improve insulin sensitivity. Further studies could shed light on ginger's potential role in managing diabetes and preventing complications.

- *Mental health:* Researchers are exploring ginger's potential in treating mental health disorders, such as depression and anxiety, by examining its effects on neurotransmitters and inflammation.

14.2 Agriculture and Plant Breeding

Advancements in agriculture and plant breeding may lead to the development of new ginger varieties with improved characteristics, such as:

- *Disease resistance:* Developing ginger varieties that are resistant to common pests and diseases could reduce crop losses and minimize the use of chemical pesticides.
- *Climate resilience:* Breeding ginger plants that can withstand changing climate conditions, such as temperature fluctuations and drought, may help ensure a stable supply of ginger in the face of climate change.
- *Enhanced nutritional and medicinal properties:* Researchers may develop ginger varieties with increased levels of bioactive compounds, offering greater health benefits and expanding its potential applications.

14.3 Biotechnology and Genetic Engineering

Biotechnology and genetic engineering could play a role in unlocking ginger's full potential by:

- _Identifying and isolating beneficial genes:_ Researchers can study ginger's genome to identify specific genes responsible for its medicinal properties, paving the way for targeted breeding programs or the development of genetically modified (GM) ginger varieties.
- _Developing GM ginger with enhanced properties:_ Genetic engineering techniques may be used to create ginger plants with improved characteristics, such as increased yield, enhanced nutritional content, or resistance to pests and diseases.

14.4 Sustainability and Circular Economy

Ginger's potential applications extend beyond its traditional uses, with researchers exploring innovative ways to utilize ginger waste and by-products in a circular economy model. Potential applications include:

- _Biofuel production:_ Converting ginger waste into biofuel could provide a renewable energy source while reducing waste disposal issues.
- _Biodegradable packaging:_ Researchers are investigating the potential of using ginger waste fibers to create biodegradable packaging materials, offering an eco-friendly alternative to traditional plastic packaging.
- _Nutraceuticals and functional foods:_ The extraction of valuable compounds from ginger waste for use in nutraceuticals and functional foods could help reduce waste while providing additional health benefits to consumers.

The future of ginger is filled with exciting possibilities, as researchers and innovators continue to explore its potential applications across various fields. Through ongoing research and development, ginger's role in medicine, agriculture, technology, and sustainability is likely to expand, further solidifying its status as a versatile and valuable plant.

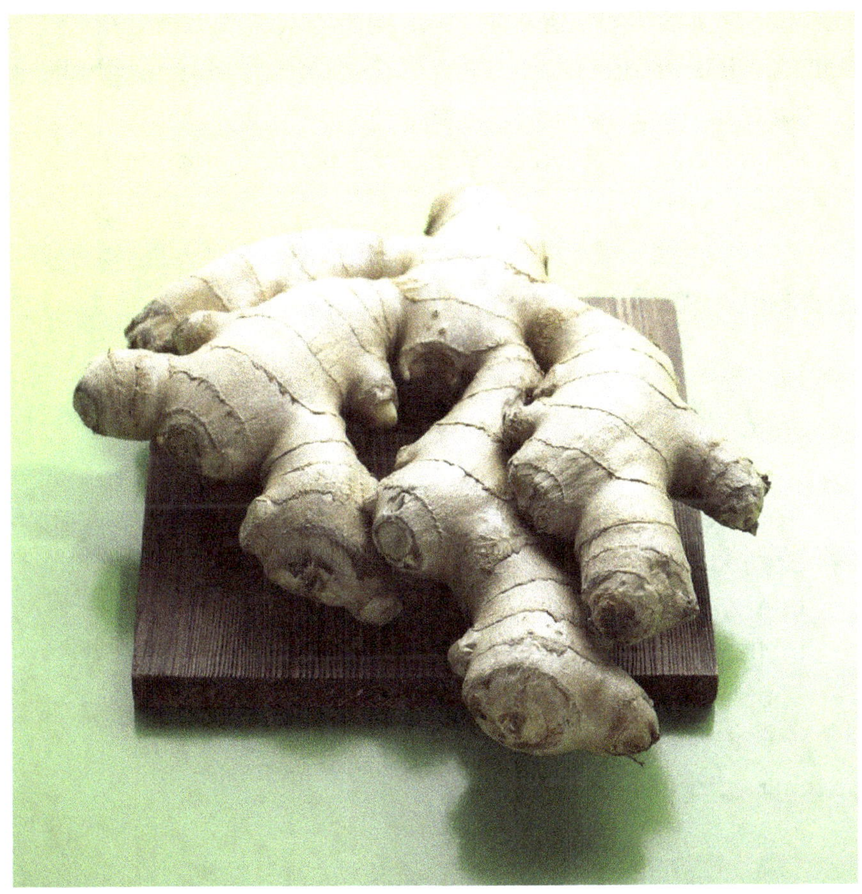

Chapter 15: The Ginger Challenge: Integrating Ginger into Your Daily Life

By now, you have discovered the incredible benefits and uses of ginger, from its medicinal properties to its culinary applications. In this final chapter, we will present the Ginger Challenge, a guide to help you incorporate ginger into your daily life, reaping its many benefits and discovering new ways to enjoy this amazing plant.

15.1 Start with Small Changes

Begin by incorporating ginger into your routine with small changes that are easy to maintain. Some ideas include:

- Add a slice of fresh ginger to your morning tea or water.
- Sprinkle ground ginger into your morning oatmeal, smoothie, or yogurt.
- Include ginger in your regular cooking, such as in stir-fries, soups, or salad dressings.

15.2 Explore New Recipes

As you become more comfortable using ginger, expand your culinary horizons by trying new recipes featuring ginger as a main ingredient. Experiment with dishes from various cuisines, such as:

- Indian curries and chutneys.
- Chinese stir-fries and dumplings.
- Japanese pickled ginger and sushi.
- Thai ginger soup (Tom Kha Gai) and salads.

15.3 Make Ginger Beverages a Part of Your Routine

Ginger beverages offer a delicious and convenient way to enjoy the benefits of ginger. Incorporate ginger drinks into your daily routine by:

- Brewing ginger tea, either from fresh ginger or store-bought tea bags.
- Making ginger lemonade or ginger-infused water for a refreshing summer drink.
- Creating ginger-based cocktails or mocktails for social gatherings or special occasions.

15.4 Incorporate Ginger into Your Health and Wellness Regimen

Explore ginger's potential health benefits by incorporating it into your wellness routine:

- Take ginger supplements or consume ginger in natural forms to help with digestion, reduce inflammation, or manage nausea.
- Use ginger essential oil in aromatherapy, massage, or as a natural remedy for colds and respiratory issues.
- Apply ginger-infused skincare products, such as masks, creams, or scrubs, for their potential antioxidant and anti-inflammatory benefits.

15.5 Spread the Word about Ginger

Share your newfound knowledge and passion for ginger with friends and family:

- Host a ginger-themed dinner party, showcasing your favorite ginger recipes.
- Gift ginger products, such as teas, spices, or skincare items, to introduce others to the benefits of ginger.
- Share articles, research, and personal experiences with ginger on social media or in conversations, helping to raise awareness of this versatile plant.

By taking on the Ginger Challenge and integrating ginger into your daily life, you'll not only enjoy its unique flavor and health benefits but also discover a newfound appreciation for this extraordinary plant. Embrace the power of ginger, and let it become a staple in your kitchen, wellness routine, and lifestyle.

Conclusion: The Lasting Impact of Ginger on Health, Wellness, and Culture

Throughout this book, we have journeyed through the fascinating world of ginger, exploring its history, cultivation, and diverse applications in medicine, cuisine, and daily life. As we reach the conclusion, it's important to reflect on the lasting impact of ginger on health, wellness, and culture, emphasizing its relevance and significance in today's world.

Ginger's well-documented medicinal properties, from reducing inflammation and easing digestive issues to potentially aiding in the management of chronic conditions, make it an invaluable addition to our health and wellness routines. As research into ginger's benefits continues, we can expect even more discoveries, solidifying its status as a powerful natural remedy. The versatility of ginger in the culinary world cannot be overstated. With its unique flavor profile and ability to enhance a wide range of dishes, ginger has earned a prominent place in kitchens around the globe. By exploring new recipes and techniques, we can continue to enjoy the vibrant taste of ginger and share it with others, contributing to a richer and more diverse global culinary landscape.

Ginger's impact on culture is also significant, as it has played a role in traditional medicine, religious practices, and trade for centuries. By understanding and appreciating ginger's cultural significance, we can gain insight into the lives and customs of those who have valued this remarkable plant throughout history.

As we move forward, the future of ginger appears bright, with ongoing research, innovations, and potential applications in various fields. By embracing ginger's many benefits and incorporating it into our daily lives, we can contribute to a healthier, more sustainable, and culturally rich world.

In conclusion, the lasting impact of ginger on health, wellness, and culture is undeniable. As you continue on your journey with ginger, may it inspire you to explore new possibilities, share its benefits with others, and appreciate the powerful legacy of this extraordinary plant.

Disclaimer:

The information contained in „Ginger (The Secrets of a Powerful Root)" is intended for educational and informational purposes only. The author and publisher are not responsible for any specific health, allergy, or medical issues that may arise from the use of the information in this book.

The author and publisher have made every effort to ensure the accuracy and completeness of the information presented in this book. However, they cannot guarantee that the information is without error or up-to-date with the latest scientific research. The reader is advised to consult with a healthcare professional before making any changes to their diet, lifestyle, or medical treatments based on the content of this book.

The suggestions and recommendations provided in this book are not intended to diagnose, treat, cure, or prevent any disease or health condition. Always seek the advice of a qualified healthcare provider with any questions you may have regarding a medical condition or any health concerns.

The author and publisher shall not be held liable for any loss, damage, or injury resulting from the use or misuse of the information in this book, nor for any actions or decisions taken by the reader based on the content herein. The reader assumes full responsibility for their actions and choices when using the information provided in this book.

Other books by the author

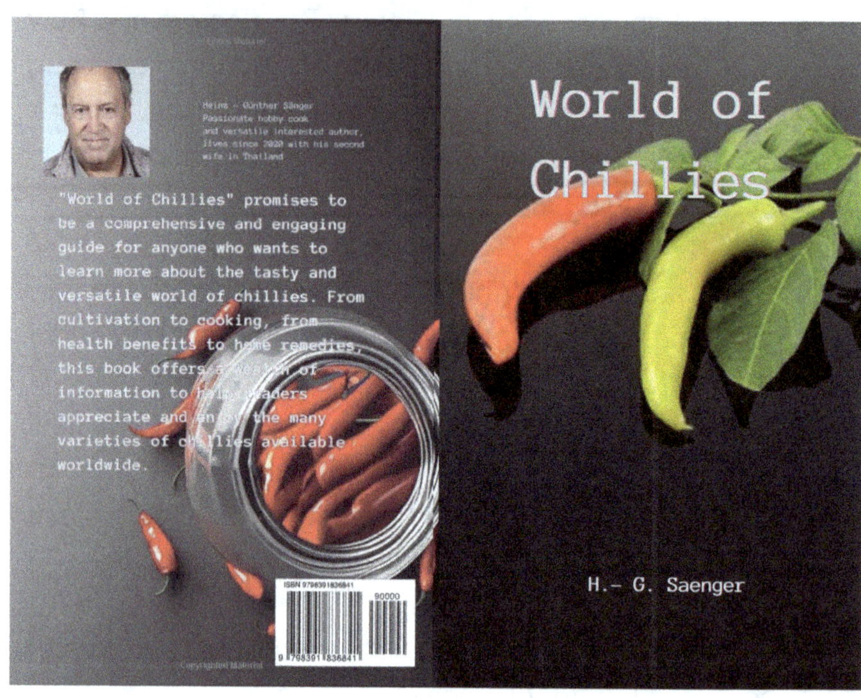

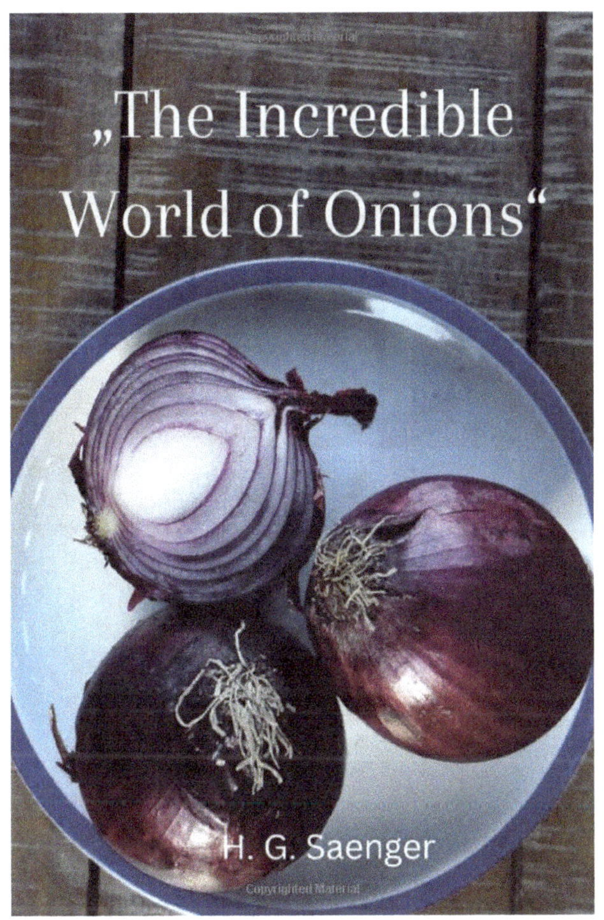
„The Incredible
World of Onions"
H. G. Saenger

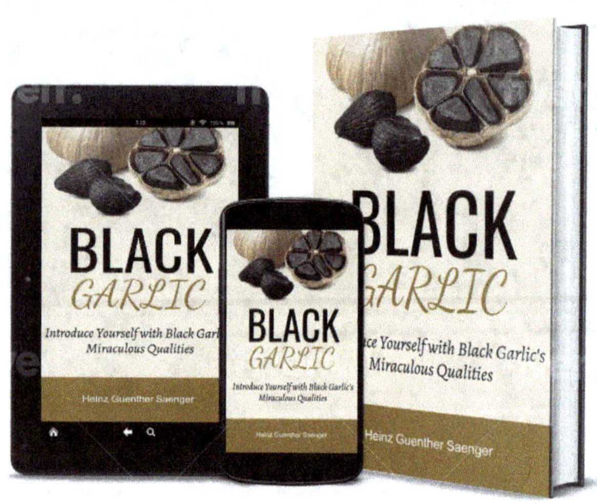

BLACK
GARLIC
Introduce Yourself with Black Garlic's
Miraculous Qualities
Heinz Guenther Saenger

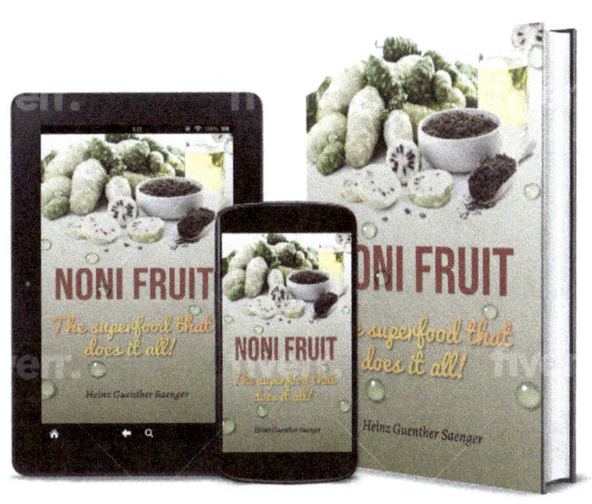
NONI FRUIT
The superfood that does it all!
Heinz Guenther Saenger

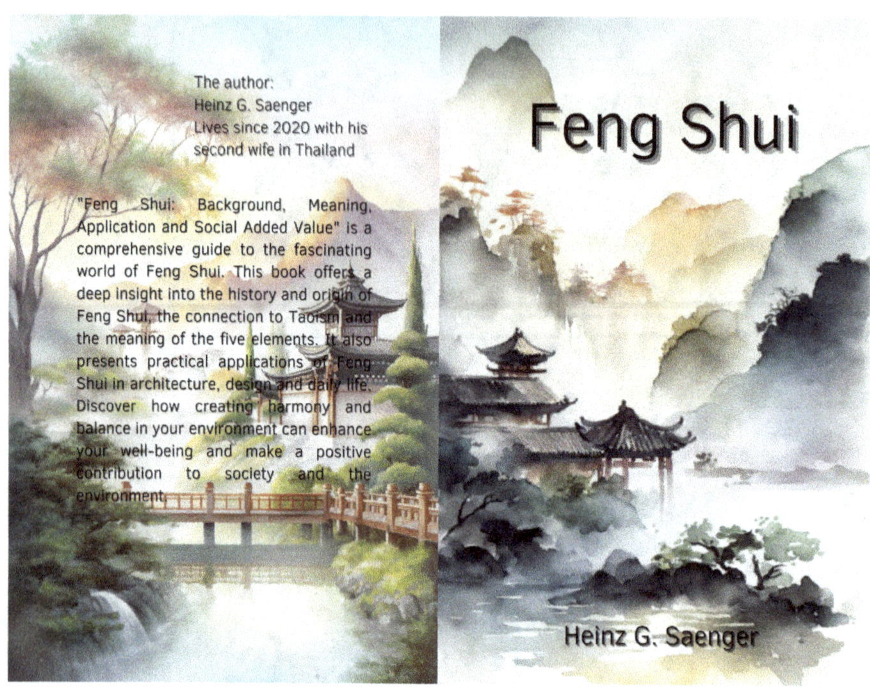
The author:
Heinz G. Saenger
Lives since 2020 with his
second wife in Thailand

"Feng Shui: Background, Meaning,
Application and Social Added Value" is a
comprehensive guide to the fascinating
world of Feng Shui. This book offers a
deep insight into the history and origin of
Feng Shui, the connection to Taoism and
the meaning of the five elements. It also
presents practical applications of Feng
Shui in architecture, design and daily life.
Discover how creating harmony and
balance in your environment can enhance
your well-being and make a positive
contribution to society and the
environment.
Feng Shui
Heinz G. Saenger

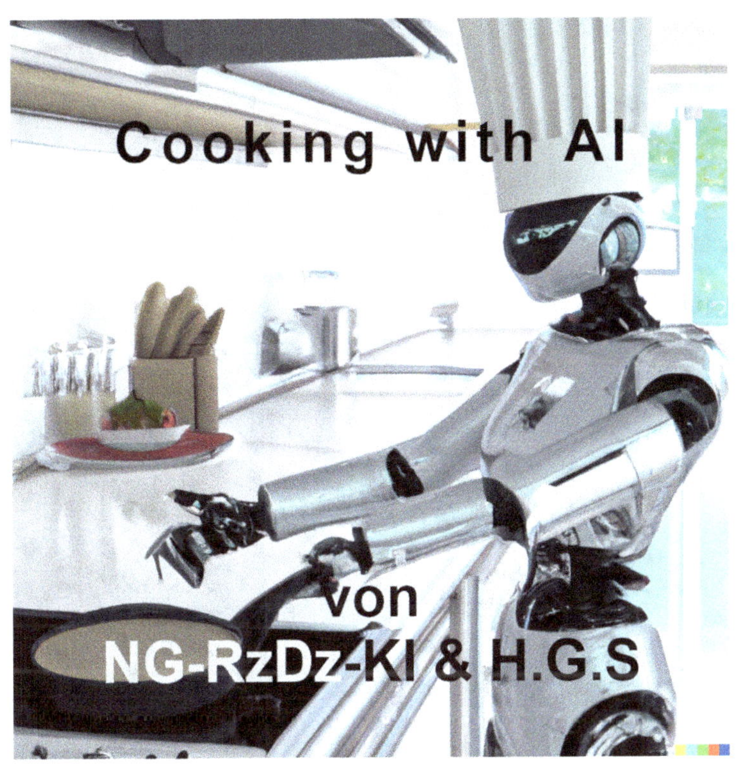

Cooking with AI
von
NG-RzDz-KI & H.G.S

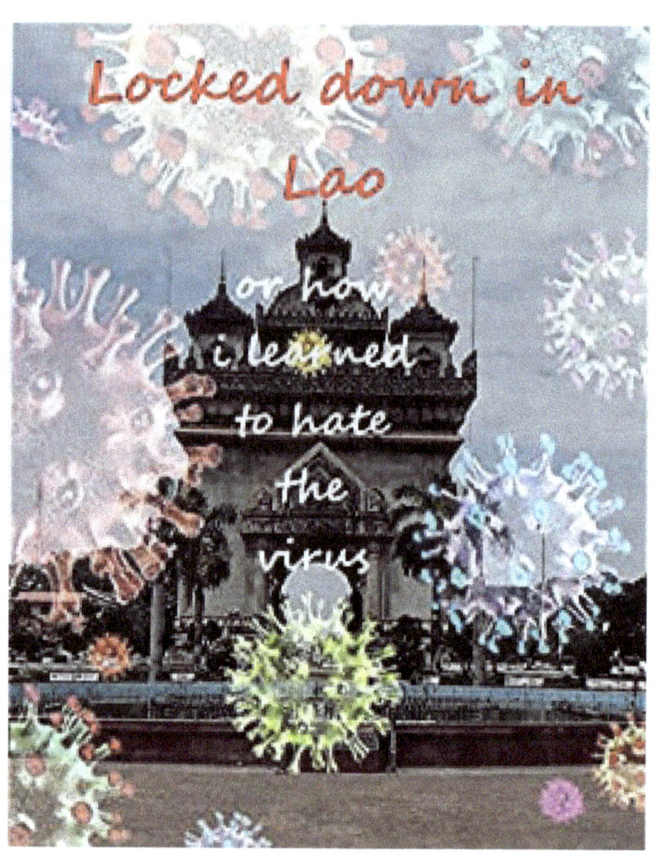

Locked down in
Lao
or how
i learned
to hate
the
virus

H. - G. Saenger

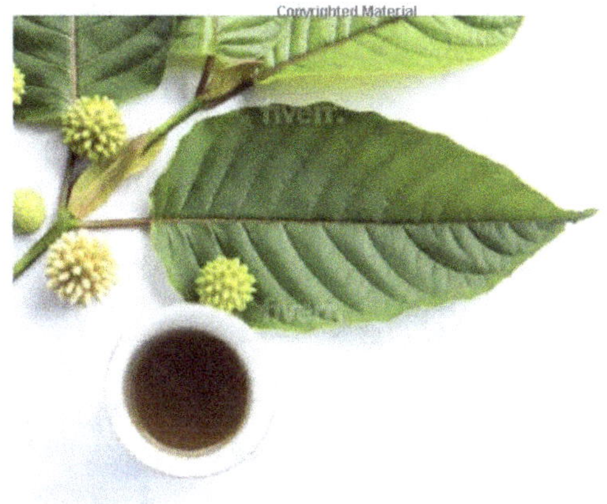

KRATOM FOR NEWBIES

All You Need To Know About Kratom Usage

By *Heinz Guenther Saenger*

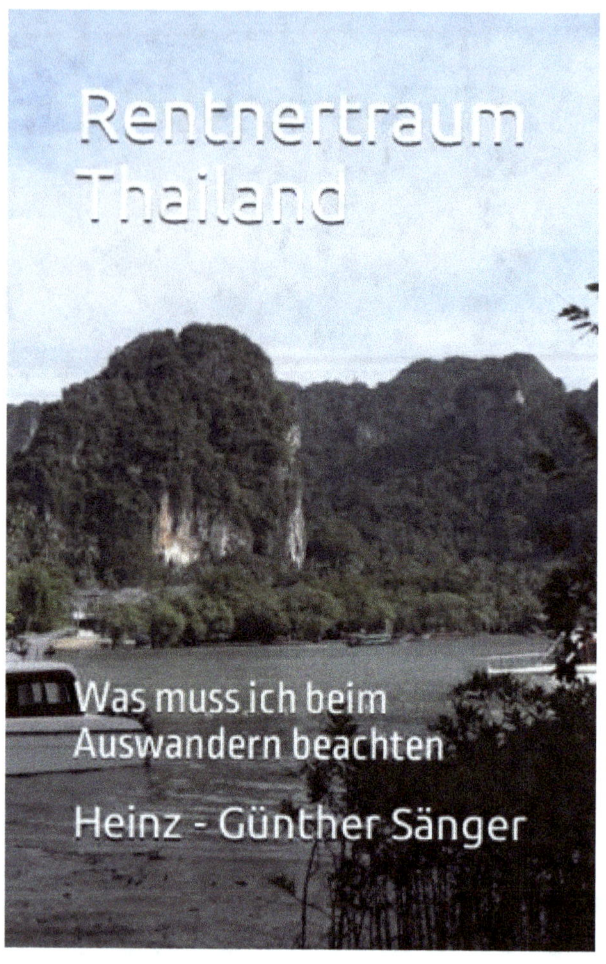

Rentnertraum
Thailand
Was muss ich beim
Auswandern beachten
Heinz - Günther Sänger

H. - G. Saenger